Unlocking the Power of Strength Training for Women: A Comprehensive Guide to Building a Lean and Fit Physique

*Empowering Women to Sculpt
Their Ideal Bodies Through
Science-Based Training and
Nutrition Strategies*

Scott Williams

Table of contents

Appreciation

Dear Readers,

As I sit down to express my gratitude, words fail to capture the depth of appreciation I feel for each and every one of you. Your support, encouragement, and enthusiasm for "Thinner Leaner Stronger: The Simple Science of Building the Ultimate Female Body" have been nothing short of incredible.

From the moment I embarked on this journey to share the science-backed principles of fitness and strength training with women everywhere, I knew that I was not alone. Your unwavering dedication to improving yourselves, both physically and mentally, has inspired me beyond measure.

It is your commitment to embracing the challenges, pushing through the obstacles, and celebrating the victories, big and small, that truly embody the spirit of Thinner Leaner Stronger. Your willingness to trust in the process, to persevere when faced with setbacks, and to uplift one another along the way, is a testament to the incredible community we have built together.

I am humbled by the countless stories of transformation, resilience, and triumph that you have shared with me. Each journey is unique, yet woven together by a common thread of strength, determination, and self-discovery. Your courage to step outside of your comfort zones, to embrace the unfamiliar, and to embrace the journey of self-improvement is nothing short of awe-inspiring.

As we continue to strive towards our goals, let us never forget the power of community, support, and camaraderie that we have cultivated together. Let us continue to lift each other up, to celebrate our successes, and to learn and grow from our experiences.

Thank you, from the bottom of my heart, for being a part of this incredible journey. Together, we are stronger, healthier, and more empowered than ever before.

With deepest gratitude,
Scott Williams

Introduction

Welcome to the world of "Thinner Leaner Stronger: The Simple Science of Building the Ultimate Female Body." In the pages that follow, you will embark on a journey that transcends the typical fitness guide, offering not just workouts and meal plans, but a comprehensive roadmap to transforming your body, mind, and life.

As a fitness enthusiast, coach, and author, I have dedicated my life to understanding the science behind building a strong, healthy, and aesthetically pleasing physique. Over the years, I have witnessed firsthand the transformative power of strength training and proper nutrition, not only in my own life but in the lives of countless women around the world.

The inspiration for "Thinner Leaner Stronger" stems from a simple yet profound belief: that every woman has the potential to sculpt her ideal body, regardless of age, fitness level, or background. Armed with the right knowledge, tools, and mindset, you can achieve results that surpass your wildest expectations.

But before we dive into the specifics of training programs, macronutrient ratios, and supplementation protocols, it's essential to lay down the foundation upon which "Thinner Leaner Stronger" is built: the science.

Understanding the Science

At the heart of "Thinner Leaner Stronger" lies a deep respect for scientific principles. Far from relying on fads, trends, or gimmicks, this book is grounded in evidence-based research, peer-reviewed studies, and real-world results. From the physiology of muscle growth to the mechanics of fat loss, every recommendation put forth in these pages is backed by solid scientific evidence.

But don't let the word "science" intimidate you. While I am passionate about the intricacies of metabolic pathways and hormonal regulation, my goal is not to overwhelm you with technical jargon or complex theories. Instead, I strive to distill the most relevant and practical information into straightforward, actionable advice that you can apply to your own life.

The Three Pillars of Success

To achieve lasting results, "Thinner Leaner Stronger" focuses on what I call the Three Pillars of Success: Training, Nutrition, and Mindset. These pillars form the cornerstone of your journey towards a stronger, leaner, and healthier body, providing a holistic approach that addresses both the physical and psychological aspects of fitness.

Training: Central to the Thinner Leaner Stronger philosophy is the belief in the transformative power of strength training. Unlike traditional cardio-centric approaches, which often lead to stagnation and frustration, strength training offers a sustainable path to long-term success. By challenging your muscles with progressively heavier weights, you will stimulate growth, increase metabolic rate, and sculpt a lean, toned physique.

Throughout this book, you will discover proven training principles, effective workout routines, and advanced techniques designed to maximize muscle growth and strength gains. Whether you're a beginner just starting out or an experienced lifter looking to take your training to the next level, there's something here for everyone.

Nutrition: They say abs are made in the kitchen, and for good reason. No amount of exercise can outwork a poor diet. That's why "Thinner Leaner Stronger" places a strong emphasis on the importance of nutrition in achieving your fitness goals. From calculating your caloric needs to understanding macronutrient ratios, you will learn how to fuel your body for optimal performance, recovery, and fat loss.

But nutrition is about more than just numbers on a scale. It's about nourishing your body with whole, nutrient-dense foods that support your health and vitality. Throughout this book, you will find practical tips, delicious recipes, and meal plans designed to make healthy eating enjoyable and sustainable.

Mindset: Last but certainly not least, "Thinner Leaner Stronger" addresses the often-overlooked element of mindset. Your mindset is the lens through which you view the world, and it plays a critical role in determining your success or failure.

By cultivating a positive, resilient mindset, you will overcome obstacles, stay motivated in the face of adversity, and unleash your full potential.

In the pages that follow, you will discover powerful mindset strategies, proven techniques for overcoming self-doubt and negative self-talk, and practical tools for staying focused and motivated on your journey. Because ultimately, it's not just about transforming your body; it's about transforming your life.

Conclusion

As you embark on this journey with me, I encourage you to approach it with an open mind, a willing heart, and a fierce determination to succeed. "Thinner Leaner Stronger" is more than just a book; it's a roadmap to a better, stronger, and more empowered version of yourself.

So, are you ready to unlock your full potential, unleash your inner strength, and build the ultimate female body? If so, let's dive in and begin this transformational journey together. Your best self awaits.

Let's make it happen.

Chapter 1: The Science of Strength Training

Welcome to Chapter 1 of "Thinner Leaner Stronger: The Simple Science of Building the Ultimate Female Body." In this chapter, we'll dive deep into the science behind strength training, exploring why it's the foundation of your fitness journey and how it can transform your body in ways you never thought possible.

The Strength Training Revolution

Strength training, once relegated to the realm of bodybuilders and athletes, has undergone a revolution in recent years. No longer seen as just a means to build muscle or increase strength, it is now recognized as one of the most effective tools for achieving a lean, toned physique, improving overall health, and enhancing quality of life.

But what exactly is strength training? At its core, strength training involves performing exercises that challenge your muscles against resistance, whether that be in the form of free weights, machines, resistance bands, or bodyweight. By subjecting your muscles to this stress, you stimulate the process of muscle growth, known as hypertrophy, leading to increases in muscle size, strength, and definition.

Contrary to popular belief, strength training is not just for men. In fact, women stand to benefit just as much, if not more, from incorporating strength training into their fitness routine. From boosting metabolism and burning fat to improving bone density and reducing the risk of injury, the benefits of strength training for women are vast and far-reaching.

The Science of Muscle Growth

To understand why strength training is so effective, it's essential to delve into the science of muscle growth. When you perform resistance exercises, you create microscopic tears in your muscle fibers. In response to this damage, your body initiates a process called muscle protein synthesis, whereby new proteins are synthesized to repair and rebuild the damaged muscle fibers.

Over time, with consistent training and proper nutrition, these repaired muscle fibers grow larger and stronger, leading to increases in muscle size and strength. This phenomenon is known as muscular adaptation, and it is the driving force behind the transformative effects of strength training.

But muscle growth is not just about lifting weights; it's also about creating the right environment within your body to support that growth. This involves ensuring adequate protein intake to provide the building blocks for muscle repair and synthesis, as well as optimizing factors such as hormone levels, sleep quality, and stress management.

The Myth of Bulking

One of the most common misconceptions surrounding strength training, particularly among women, is the fear of getting bulky. Many women worry that lifting heavy weights will cause them to develop large, bulky muscles, leading to a less feminine appearance.

However, this fear is unfounded. Unlike men, who have significantly higher levels of testosterone, the hormone primarily responsible for muscle growth, women have much lower levels, making it much more difficult for them to bulk up. In fact, most women lack the genetic predisposition to develop large, bulky muscles, even with intense strength training.

Instead, what women can expect from strength training is a lean, toned physique characterized by sculpted muscles and a defined silhouette. By focusing on moderate to heavy weights and higher rep ranges, women can achieve the perfect balance of muscle tone and definition without fear of bulking up.

The Importance of Progressive Overload

Key to the success of any strength training program is the principle of progressive overload. This principle states that in order for muscles to grow and adapt, they must be subjected to progressively greater levels of stress over time. This can be achieved by increasing the weight lifted, the number of repetitions performed, or the intensity of the workout.

By continually challenging your muscles in this way, you force them to adapt and grow stronger, leading to ongoing improvements in muscle size, strength, and definition. Without progressive overload, your muscles would quickly plateau, and your progress would stagnate.

Designing Your Strength Training Program

Now that you understand the science behind strength training, it's time to put that knowledge into action by designing your own personalized strength training program. This program will serve as the blueprint for your fitness journey, guiding you through a series of workouts designed to maximize muscle growth, strength gains, and fat loss.

But before we dive into the specifics of program design, it's essential to establish clear goals and objectives for your training. Whether your goal is to build muscle, increase strength, or lose fat, having a clear vision of what you want to achieve will help you tailor your program to suit your needs and preferences.

In the next chapter, we'll explore the fundamentals of program design, including exercise selection, set and rep schemes, and training frequency, to help

you create a program that aligns with your goals
and maximizes your results.

Conclusion

In conclusion, strength training is not just a means
to build muscle or increase strength; it's a powerful
tool for transforming your body, mind, and life. By
understanding the science behind strength training
and applying the principles of progressive overload,
you can unlock your full potential and achieve the
lean, toned physique you've always dreamed of.

In the next chapter, we'll dive into the nitty-gritty
details of program design, helping you create a
customized strength training program that will set
you on the path to success. So, are you ready to
take the first step towards a stronger, leaner, and
more empowered you? Let's do this.

Chapter 2: Designing Your Strength Training Program

Welcome to Chapter 2 of "Thinner Leaner Stronger: The Simple Science of Building the Ultimate Female Body." In this chapter, we'll delve into the fundamentals of program design, equipping you with the knowledge and tools you need to create a customized strength training program that will maximize your results and propel you towards your fitness goals.

Setting Clear Goals

Before we jump into the specifics of program design, it's essential to establish clear and achievable goals for your strength training journey. Whether your goal is to build muscle, increase strength, improve athletic performance, or lose fat, having a clear understanding of what you want to achieve will help guide your training and keep you motivated along the way.

When setting goals, it's important to make them specific, measurable, achievable, relevant, and time-bound (SMART). For example, rather than simply saying, "I want to build muscle," a SMART goal might be, "I want to increase my lean muscle mass by 5% within the next six months."

By setting SMART goals, you give yourself a clear target to aim for and a deadline to work towards, increasing your motivation and accountability in the process.

Exercise Selection

Once you've established your goals, the next step is to choose the exercises that will form the foundation of your strength training program. When selecting exercises, it's important to focus on compound movements that engage multiple muscle groups simultaneously, such as squats, deadlifts, bench presses, rows, and overhead presses.

Compound exercises not only allow you to lift heavier weights and build more muscle mass but also provide functional benefits that carry over into everyday activities and sports performance. Additionally, by incorporating compound movements into your program, you can maximize efficiency and time effectiveness, as these exercises target multiple muscle groups with each repetition.

In addition to compound exercises, you may also choose to include isolation exercises to target specific muscle groups or address individual weaknesses or imbalances. Examples of isolation exercises include bicep curls, tricep extensions, lateral raises, and leg curls.

Set and Rep Schemes

Once you've selected your exercises, the next step is to determine the set and rep schemes that will comprise each workout. Set and rep schemes refer to the number of sets and repetitions performed for each exercise and play a critical role in determining the intensity and volume of your workouts.

There are numerous set and rep schemes to choose from, each with its own unique benefits and applications. Some common examples include:

- **Straight Sets:** Performing a fixed number of repetitions for a specified number of sets, with the same weight for each set.
- **Pyramid Sets:** Gradually increasing or decreasing the weight lifted with each set, while maintaining a consistent number of repetitions.
- **Supersets:** Alternating between two different exercises, typically targeting opposing muscle groups, with minimal rest between sets.
- **Drop Sets:** Performing a set of an exercise to failure, then immediately reducing the weight and continuing to perform additional repetitions until failure is reached again.
- **Circuit Training:** Performing a series of exercises in rapid succession, with minimal rest between exercises, to increase cardiovascular conditioning and calorie burn.

The optimal set and rep scheme for you will depend on your individual goals, preferences, and training experience. Experiment with different schemes to find what works best for you, and don't be afraid to adjust your program as needed based on your progress and feedback.

Training Frequency

Another key consideration when designing your strength training program is training frequency, or how often you should train each muscle group per week. While there is no one-size-fits-all answer to this question, as individual responses to training can vary widely, there are some general guidelines that can help you determine the optimal training frequency for your goals.

For beginners, it's typically recommended to start with a lower training frequency, such as two to three times per week per muscle group, to allow for adequate recovery and adaptation. As you become more experienced and your recovery capacity improves, you may choose to increase your training frequency to four or even five times per week per muscle group.

It's important to listen to your body and pay attention to signs of overtraining, such as persistent fatigue, soreness, or lack of progress. If you find yourself experiencing these symptoms, consider reducing your training frequency or increasing your rest days to allow for proper recovery and avoid burnout.

Progressive Overload and Periodization

At the heart of any effective strength training program is the principle of progressive overload, which we discussed in Chapter 1. Progressive overload refers to the gradual increase in training stimulus over time to continue driving adaptations in muscle size, strength, and performance.

There are many ways to implement progressive overload into your training program, including:

- Increasing the weight lifted
- Increasing the number of repetitions performed
- Increasing the number of sets performed
- Decreasing rest periods between sets
- Varying the tempo or speed of each repetition
- Incorporating advanced training techniques, such as rest-pause sets, drop sets, or forced reps

In addition to progressive overload, another important concept in program design is periodization, which involves dividing your training program into distinct phases or cycles, each with its own specific focus and objectives. By varying the intensity, volume, and exercise selection throughout each phase, periodization helps prevent plateaus, reduce the risk of overtraining, and optimize long-term progress and performance.

Conclusion

In conclusion, designing an effective strength training program requires careful consideration of a variety of factors, including your goals, exercise selection, set and rep schemes, training frequency, and progressive overload strategies. By taking the time to plan and structure your workouts thoughtfully, you can maximize your results and achieve your desired outcomes more efficiently and effectively.

In the next chapter, we'll explore the practical application of these principles by providing sample workout routines and templates that you can use to kickstart your strength training journey. Whether you're a beginner just starting out or an experienced lifter looking to take your training to the next level, there's something here for everyone.

So, are you ready to design the ultimate strength training program that will transform your body and elevate your fitness to new heights? Let's get started.

Chapter 3: Nutrition Essentials for Strength Training Success

Welcome to Chapter 3 of "Thinner Leaner Stronger: The Simple Science of Building the Ultimate Female Body." In this chapter, we'll explore the essential role that nutrition plays in supporting your strength training efforts and maximizing your results. From fueling your workouts to optimizing recovery and promoting muscle growth, nutrition is a critical component of any successful fitness journey.

Understanding Macronutrients

Before we dive into the specifics of nutrition for strength training, let's start by examining the three macronutrients that make up the bulk of your diet: protein, carbohydrates, and fats.

- **Protein:** Often referred to as the building blocks of muscle, protein plays a crucial role in repairing and rebuilding muscle tissue damaged during exercise. Aim to consume a sufficient amount of high-quality protein sources, such as lean meats, poultry, fish, eggs, dairy products, legumes, and tofu, to support muscle growth and repair.

- **Carbohydrates:** Carbohydrates serve as the primary fuel source for high-intensity exercise, providing your muscles with the energy they need to perform optimally during workouts. Focus on consuming complex carbohydrates, such as whole grains, fruits, vegetables, and legumes, which provide sustained energy and essential nutrients.

- **Fats:** Despite their often-maligned reputation, fats are an essential nutrient that plays a variety of roles in the body, including hormone production, cell membrane integrity, and nutrient absorption. Opt for healthy fats, such as those found in avocados, nuts, seeds, olive oil, and fatty fish, while minimizing intake of trans fats and saturated fats.

By understanding the unique roles that each macronutrient plays in supporting your training and recovery, you can optimize your diet to fuel your workouts, enhance performance, and achieve your fitness goals more effectively.

Caloric Intake and Macronutrient Ratios

In addition to understanding the importance of individual macronutrients, it's also essential to consider your overall caloric intake and macronutrient ratios when designing your nutrition plan.

Caloric intake refers to the total number of calories you consume each day, while macronutrient ratios refer to the proportion of calories that come from each macronutrient. The optimal caloric intake and macronutrient ratios for you will depend on factors such as your age, gender, weight, height, activity level, and fitness goals.

For example, if your goal is to build muscle and increase strength, you may need to consume a slight caloric surplus to provide your body with the energy it needs to support muscle growth and repair. In terms of macronutrient ratios, a typical recommendation for strength training is to consume approximately 1.2 to 2.2 grams of protein per kilogram of body weight, 3 to 6 grams of carbohydrates per kilogram of body weight, and 0.5 to 1 gram of fat per kilogram of body weight per day.

However, it's important to note that these are just general guidelines, and individual needs may vary. Experiment with different caloric intakes and macronutrient ratios to find what works best for you, and consider seeking guidance from a registered dietitian or nutritionist for personalized recommendations.

Meal Timing and Composition

In addition to total caloric intake and macronutrient ratios, meal timing and composition also play a role in optimizing performance, recovery, and muscle growth. Aim to consume a balanced meal or snack containing protein, carbohydrates, and fats approximately 1 to 3 hours before your workout to provide your body with the energy it needs to perform at its best.

After your workout, prioritize consuming a meal or snack containing a combination of protein and carbohydrates within 30 to 60 minutes to replenish glycogen stores, repair muscle tissue, and promote recovery. This post-workout meal, often referred to as the "anabolic window," is a critical time for nutrient delivery and muscle repair, so be sure to prioritize it in your nutrition plan.

Throughout the rest of the day, aim to spread your meals and snacks evenly across the day to provide your body with a steady stream of nutrients and energy. This can help regulate blood sugar levels, prevent energy crashes, and optimize metabolism and digestion.

Supplements for Strength Training

While proper nutrition should always be the foundation of your diet, supplements can also play a role in supporting your strength training efforts and enhancing performance, recovery, and muscle growth. Some common supplements used by strength trainers include:

- **Whey Protein:** A convenient and easily digestible source of protein, whey protein can help meet your daily protein needs and support muscle recovery and growth.

- **Creatine:** One of the most extensively researched supplements for strength and muscle building, creatine has been shown to increase muscle mass, strength, and exercise performance.

- **BCAAs (Branched-Chain Amino Acids):** Comprising the essential amino acids leucine, isoleucine, and valine, BCAAs can help reduce muscle soreness, enhance recovery, and preserve lean muscle mass during periods of calorie restriction or intense training.

While supplements can be beneficial, it's important to remember that they are not a substitute for a healthy, balanced diet. Always prioritize whole foods first, and use supplements as a complement to fill any nutritional gaps or enhance specific aspects of your training and recovery.

Nutrition for Fat Loss

In addition to supporting muscle growth and strength gains, nutrition also plays a critical role in fat loss and body composition. By creating a caloric deficit, or consuming fewer calories than you expend, you can force your body to tap into stored fat reserves for energy, leading to fat loss over time.

However, it's important to create a modest caloric deficit and prioritize nutrient-dense foods to ensure that you still meet your body's nutritional needs and support overall health and well-being. Aim to consume a balance of protein, carbohydrates, and fats, while focusing on whole, minimally processed foods that provide essential vitamins, minerals, and antioxidants.

In addition to creating a caloric deficit, other strategies that can support fat loss include increasing protein intake to promote satiety and preserve lean muscle mass, incorporating strength training to maintain metabolic rate and promote fat oxidation, and prioritizing sleep, stress management, and hydration to optimize metabolism and hormone balance.

Conclusion

In conclusion, nutrition is a critical component of strength training success, providing the fuel your body needs to perform optimally, recover effectively, and achieve your fitness goals. By understanding the roles of macronutrients, optimizing caloric intake and macronutrient ratios, timing your meals strategically, and incorporating supplements as needed, you can create a nutrition plan that supports your strength training efforts and maximizes your results.

In the next chapter, we'll put theory into practice by providing sample meal plans and recipes that you can use to fuel your workouts, support your recovery, and optimize your performance in the gym. Whether your goal is to build muscle, increase strength, or lose fat, these practical nutrition strategies will help you achieve your desired outcomes and unlock your full potential.

So, are you ready to take your nutrition to the next level and fuel your journey towards a stronger, leaner, and more empowered you? Let's dive in and make it happen.

Chapter 4: Practical Nutrition Strategies for Strength Training Success

Welcome to Chapter 4 of "Thinner Leaner Stronger: The Simple Science of Building the Ultimate Female Body." In this chapter, we'll translate the principles of nutrition into practical strategies that you can implement in your daily life to fuel your strength training journey, support your recovery, and optimize your performance in the gym.

Creating Balanced Meal Plans

One of the most effective ways to ensure that you're meeting your nutritional needs and fueling your workouts properly is to create balanced meal plans that prioritize whole, nutrient-dense foods. A balanced meal plan typically includes a combination of lean protein sources, complex carbohydrates, healthy fats, fruits, vegetables, and plenty of water.

When designing your meal plan, aim to include a variety of foods from each food group to ensure that you're getting a wide range of essential nutrients and micronutrients. For example, you might start your day with a breakfast of Greek yogurt topped with fresh fruit and nuts, followed by a lunch of grilled chicken with quinoa and roasted vegetables, and finish with a dinner of salmon with sweet potatoes and steamed broccoli.

In addition to main meals, be sure to include snacks throughout the day to keep your energy levels stable and prevent overeating at meal times.

Healthy snack options might include a handful of almonds and an apple, a protein smoothie made with whey protein powder and berries, or a serving of Greek yogurt with granola.

Meal Prep and Batch Cooking

To make sticking to your meal plan easier and more convenient, consider incorporating meal prep and batch cooking into your routine. Set aside time each week to plan and prepare your meals in advance, chopping vegetables, cooking proteins, and portioning out servings into containers for easy grab-and-go access throughout the week.

By prepping your meals ahead of time, you can save time and effort during busy weekdays, minimize the temptation to reach for unhealthy convenience foods, and ensure that you have nutritious options readily available whenever hunger strikes. Plus, by cooking in bulk and freezing leftovers, you can reduce food waste and save money in the long run.

Strategic Nutrient Timing

In addition to focusing on what you eat, it's also important to consider when you eat, particularly in relation to your workouts. Strategic nutrient timing, or consuming specific nutrients at specific times before, during, and after exercise, can help optimize performance, recovery, and muscle growth.

Before your workout, aim to consume a balanced meal or snack containing carbohydrates and protein approximately 1 to 3 hours beforehand to provide your body with the energy it needs to fuel your workout and support muscle protein synthesis. Examples of pre-workout snacks might include a banana with almond butter, a turkey and cheese sandwich on whole grain bread, or a protein shake with oats and fruit.

During your workout, stay hydrated by drinking water or a sports drink to replace fluids lost through sweat and maintain optimal hydration levels. Depending on the duration and intensity of your workout, you may also benefit from consuming a small snack containing carbohydrates, such as a piece of fruit or a sports gel, to provide additional energy and prevent fatigue.

After your workout, prioritize consuming a meal or snack containing a combination of protein and carbohydrates within 30 to 60 minutes to replenish glycogen stores, repair muscle tissue, and promote recovery. This post-workout meal, often referred to as the "anabolic window," is a critical time for nutrient delivery and muscle repair, so be sure to prioritize it in your nutrition plan.

Hydration and Recovery

In addition to focusing on food, it's also important to pay attention to your hydration and recovery practices to support your strength training efforts. Adequate hydration is essential for maintaining optimal performance, preventing dehydration, and supporting overall health and well-being.

To stay hydrated throughout the day, aim to drink plenty of water and other hydrating fluids, such as herbal tea, coconut water, or diluted fruit juice. Monitor your urine color and output as a general guideline for hydration status, aiming for pale yellow urine and frequent bathroom breaks.

In addition to staying hydrated, prioritize recovery strategies such as adequate sleep, stress management, and active rest days to support muscle repair and growth, reduce the risk of overtraining, and promote overall recovery and well-being. Aim for 7-9 hours of quality sleep per night, practice relaxation techniques such as deep breathing or meditation, and incorporate light activities such as walking or yoga on rest days to promote blood flow and reduce muscle soreness.

Individualizing Your Nutrition Plan

Finally, it's important to remember that there is no one-size-fits-all approach to nutrition, and what works for one person may not work for another. Experiment with different meal plans, timing strategies, and food choices to find what works best for your body, preferences, and lifestyle.

Listen to your body's hunger and fullness cues, pay attention to how different foods make you feel, and adjust your nutrition plan accordingly based on your goals, preferences, and feedback. Consider working with a registered dietitian or nutritionist to develop a personalized nutrition plan tailored to your individual needs and goals.

Conclusion

In conclusion, nutrition is a critical component of strength training success, providing the fuel your body needs to perform optimally, recover effectively, and achieve your fitness goals. By focusing on balanced meal plans, strategic nutrient timing, hydration and recovery practices, and individualizing your nutrition plan, you can optimize your performance in the gym and maximize your results.

In the next chapter, we'll shift our focus to supplementation and explore the role that supplements can play in supporting your strength training efforts and enhancing your overall health and well-being. Whether you're looking to boost performance, improve recovery, or fill nutritional gaps in your diet, supplements can be a valuable tool in your arsenal for success.

So, are you ready to take your nutrition to the next level and fuel your journey towards a stronger, leaner, and more empowered you? Let's dive in and make it happen.

Chapter 5: Enhancing Performance and Recovery with Supplements

Welcome to Chapter 5 of "Thinner Leaner Stronger: The Simple Science of Building the Ultimate Female Body." In this chapter, we'll explore the role that supplements can play in supporting your strength training efforts, enhancing performance, and promoting recovery. From protein powders to vitamins and minerals, supplements can be a valuable tool in your arsenal for success.

Understanding Supplements

Before we dive into specific supplements, let's take a moment to understand what supplements are and how they can support your fitness goals. Supplements are products that contain one or more dietary ingredients intended to supplement the diet, such as vitamins, minerals, herbs, amino acids, or other substances.

While supplements should never replace a healthy, balanced diet, they can be used to fill nutritional gaps, enhance performance, improve recovery, and support overall health and well-being. When choosing supplements, it's important to select high-quality products from reputable brands and to use them as part of a comprehensive nutrition and training plan.

Protein Powder

One of the most popular and widely used supplements among strength trainers is protein powder. Protein powder is a convenient and easily digestible source of protein, making it an ideal option for increasing protein intake and supporting muscle growth and repair.

There are several types of protein powder available, including whey, casein, soy, pea, and rice protein, each with its own unique characteristics and benefits. Whey protein, in particular, is a fast-digesting protein that is rich in essential amino acids, making it an ideal choice for post-workout recovery.

To incorporate protein powder into your nutrition plan, simply mix a scoop of powder with water, milk, or a smoothie and consume it before or after your workout, or as a snack throughout the day. Experiment with different flavors and brands to find one that you enjoy and that fits your dietary preferences and goals.

Creatine

Another popular supplement for strength trainers is creatine. Creatine is a naturally occurring compound found in the body that plays a key role in energy production during high-intensity exercise. By supplementing with creatine, you can increase the availability of creatine phosphate in your muscles, allowing you to perform better during short, intense bursts of activity.

Research has shown that creatine supplementation can increase muscle mass, strength, power output, and exercise performance, particularly during activities that require short, explosive efforts, such as weightlifting and sprinting. Additionally, creatine has been shown to aid in recovery and reduce muscle soreness, allowing you to train harder and more frequently.

To supplement with creatine, simply mix a small dose of creatine monohydrate powder with water or juice and consume it before or after your workout. Alternatively, you can take a daily maintenance dose of creatine to saturate your muscles over time and reap the benefits of improved performance and recovery.

BCAAs (Branched-Chain Amino Acids)

BCAAs, or branched-chain amino acids, are a group of essential amino acids that include leucine, isoleucine, and valine. BCAAs are unique in that they are metabolized directly in the muscles rather than in the liver, making them readily available for energy production and muscle repair during exercise.

Supplementing with BCAAs can help reduce muscle soreness, improve recovery, and preserve lean muscle mass, particularly during periods of calorie restriction or intense training. BCAAs have also been shown to enhance endurance performance, delay fatigue, and promote fat oxidation during exercise.

To supplement with BCAAs, simply mix a scoop of BCAA powder with water and consume it before, during, or after your workout. Alternatively, you can take BCAA capsules or tablets if you prefer a more convenient option.

Omega-3 Fatty Acids

Omega-3 fatty acids are essential fats that play a variety of roles in the body, including supporting heart health, reducing inflammation, and improving brain function. Omega-3s are particularly beneficial for strength trainers due to their anti-inflammatory properties, which can help reduce muscle soreness and promote recovery after intense workouts.

Sources of omega-3 fatty acids include fatty fish such as salmon, mackerel, and sardines, as well as flaxseeds, chia seeds, and walnuts. However, many people struggle to consume enough omega-3s through diet alone, making supplementation a convenient option.

To supplement with omega-3 fatty acids, look for a high-quality fish oil or algae oil supplement that provides a concentrated dose of EPA and DHA, the two most important omega-3 fatty acids. Aim to consume around 1-2 grams of combined EPA and

DHA per day to support overall health and well-being.

Vitamins and Minerals

In addition to specific supplements targeted towards performance and recovery, it's also important to ensure that you're meeting your body's needs for essential vitamins and minerals. While a balanced diet should provide most of the vitamins and minerals you need, certain individuals may benefit from supplementation, particularly if they have specific dietary restrictions or deficiencies.

Some common vitamins and minerals that are important for strength trainers include vitamin D, calcium, magnesium, and iron. Vitamin D plays a key role in bone health and immune function, while calcium and magnesium are essential for muscle contraction and relaxation. Iron is necessary for oxygen transport and energy production, making it particularly important for endurance athletes.

If you're concerned about your vitamin and mineral intake, consider speaking with a healthcare provider or registered dietitian to determine if supplementation is necessary. They can help assess your individual needs and recommend appropriate supplements to fill any nutritional gaps in your diet.

Conclusion

In conclusion, supplements can be a valuable tool in supporting your strength training efforts, enhancing performance, and promoting recovery. From protein powder to creatine, BCAAs, omega-3 fatty acids, and vitamins and minerals, there are a variety of supplements available that can help you achieve your fitness goals more effectively.

However, it's important to remember that supplements should never replace a healthy, balanced diet, and that their effectiveness can vary depending on factors such as dosage, timing, and individual response. Always choose high-quality products from reputable brands, and use supplements as part of a comprehensive nutrition and training plan.

In the next chapter, we'll wrap up our discussion by exploring practical strategies for staying motivated, overcoming obstacles, and sustaining long-term success on your fitness journey. Whether you're just starting out or you're a seasoned strength trainer, these tips and techniques will help you stay on track and achieve your goals.

So, are you ready to take your performance and recovery to the next level with supplements? Let's dive in and make it happen.

Chapter 6: Sustaining Long-Term Success: Strategies for Motivation and Overcoming Obstacles

Welcome to Chapter 6 of "Thinner Leaner Stronger: The Simple Science of Building the Ultimate Female Body." In this chapter, we'll explore practical strategies for sustaining long-term success on your fitness journey, including tips for staying motivated, overcoming obstacles, and maintaining consistency in your training and nutrition habits.

Setting Realistic Expectations

One of the keys to long-term success in any endeavor is setting realistic expectations for yourself. While it's important to have ambitious goals and aspirations, it's equally important to recognize that progress takes time and that setbacks and obstacles are a normal part of the process.

Instead of expecting overnight results or perfection from yourself, focus on making small, sustainable changes to your habits and routines that will gradually move you closer to your goals. Celebrate your progress along the way, no matter how small, and be patient with yourself as you navigate the ups and downs of your fitness journey.

Finding Your Why

Another important factor in sustaining long-term success is identifying your "why" – the underlying reason or motivation behind your desire to improve your fitness and health. Your why is what will drive you to stay committed and focused on your goals, even when faced with challenges or setbacks.

Take some time to reflect on why you want to build a stronger, leaner body and how achieving your goals will positively impact your life. Whether it's to feel more confident, improve your health, set a positive example for others, or simply challenge yourself to be the best version of yourself, clarifying your why can help fuel your motivation and keep you on track when times get tough.

Setting SMART Goals

In addition to identifying your overarching why, it's also important to set specific, measurable, achievable, relevant, and time-bound (SMART) goals to guide your efforts and keep you accountable. SMART goals provide a clear roadmap for success and allow you to track your progress over time, making it easier to stay motivated and focused on your objectives.

When setting SMART goals, be sure to break them down into smaller, more manageable milestones or action steps that you can work towards on a daily or weekly basis. This will help prevent overwhelm and ensure that you're making consistent progress towards your ultimate vision of success.

Creating a Supportive Environment

Surrounding yourself with a supportive environment can also play a crucial role in sustaining long-term success on your fitness journey. Whether it's finding a workout buddy, joining a fitness community or support group, or enlisting the help of a coach or mentor, having a network of like-minded individuals who share your goals and values can provide invaluable encouragement, accountability, and motivation.

In addition to seeking support from others, it's also important to create an environment that supports your goals and makes it easier for you to stick to your training and nutrition habits. This might involve meal prepping and planning your workouts in advance, setting up a dedicated workout space at home, or removing temptations and distractions that could derail your progress.

Practicing Self-Compassion

Finally, it's important to practice self-compassion and kindness towards yourself as you navigate the ups and downs of your fitness journey. It's normal to experience setbacks, plateaus, and moments of doubt along the way, but beating yourself up or dwelling on negative thoughts will only make it harder to stay motivated and focused on your goals.

Instead, practice self-compassion by treating yourself with the same kindness and understanding that you would extend to a friend or loved one facing similar challenges. Focus on progress over perfection, celebrate your successes, and learn from your mistakes without dwelling on them or letting them define your self-worth.

Conclusion

In conclusion, sustaining long-term success on your fitness journey requires a combination of motivation, resilience, and consistency in your habits and routines. By setting realistic expectations, clarifying your why, setting SMART goals, creating a supportive environment, and practicing self-compassion, you can overcome obstacles, stay motivated, and achieve your goals more effectively and sustainably.

Remember that fitness is not just about reaching a destination but rather enjoying the journey and embracing the process of growth and self-improvement along the way. Stay committed, stay focused, and stay true to yourself, and you'll be amazed at what you can achieve.

In closing, I want to thank you for joining me on this journey through "Thinner Leaner Stronger: The Simple Science of Building the Ultimate Female Body." I hope that the knowledge, tools, and strategies shared in this book will empower you to take control of your fitness and health and create the strong, lean body you've always dreamed of.

Remember, you have everything you need within you to succeed. Now, go out there and make it happen.

Chapter 7: The Power of Mindset: Cultivating Mental Strength for Fitness Success

Welcome to Chapter 7 of "Thinner Leaner Stronger: The Simple Science of Building the Ultimate Female Body." In this chapter, we'll explore the importance of mindset in achieving fitness success and discuss strategies for cultivating mental strength, resilience, and positivity on your journey towards a stronger, leaner body.

The Role of Mindset in Fitness Success

While physical strength and conditioning are crucial components of achieving your fitness goals, the power of mindset cannot be overstated. Your mindset – the attitudes, beliefs, and thought patterns that shape your behavior and responses to challenges – plays a critical role in determining your success and satisfaction in any endeavor, including fitness.

A positive mindset can help you stay motivated, overcome obstacles, and bounce back from setbacks more effectively, while a negative mindset can hold you back, undermine your confidence, and sabotage your progress. By cultivating a growth-oriented mindset focused on learning, resilience, and self-improvement, you can unlock your full potential and achieve your goals more efficiently and sustainably.

Embracing the Growth Mindset

At the heart of a positive mindset is the concept of the growth mindset, popularized by psychologist Carol Dweck. A growth mindset is the belief that your abilities and intelligence can be developed through dedication and hard work, rather than being fixed traits that you either have or don't have.

Individuals with a growth mindset approach challenges and setbacks as opportunities for growth and learning, viewing failures not as evidence of their limitations but as stepping stones on the path to success. They embrace effort, persist in the face of obstacles, and seek out feedback and constructive criticism as valuable tools for improvement.

By cultivating a growth mindset in your fitness journey, you can reframe challenges as opportunities for growth, view setbacks as temporary setbacks rather than insurmountable barriers, and approach your training and nutrition with a sense of curiosity, experimentation, and resilience.

Cultivating Resilience

In addition to embracing a growth mindset, cultivating resilience – the ability to bounce back from adversity and overcome challenges – is another essential aspect of mental strength for fitness success. Resilience involves developing coping strategies, building social support networks, and practicing self-care to navigate the inevitable ups and downs of your fitness journey.

One way to cultivate resilience is to develop a toolbox of coping strategies that you can turn to when faced with challenges or setbacks. This might include techniques such as positive self-talk, visualization, deep breathing, mindfulness meditation, or seeking support from friends, family, or a coach.

Building strong social support networks can also help bolster resilience by providing encouragement, accountability, and perspective when faced with challenges. Surround yourself with positive, supportive individuals who share your goals and values, and don't hesitate to lean on them for support when needed.

Finally, practicing self-care – taking time to rest, recharge, and nurture your physical, mental, and emotional well-being – is essential for maintaining resilience and preventing burnout. Prioritize activities that bring you joy, relaxation, and fulfillment, whether it's spending time with loved ones, pursuing hobbies and interests, or simply taking a break from training to rest and recover.

Cultivating Positivity and Gratitude

In addition to embracing a growth mindset and cultivating resilience, cultivating positivity and gratitude can also help support your mental strength and well-being on your fitness journey. Positive thinking and gratitude practices have been linked to numerous psychological and physical health benefits, including reduced stress, improved mood, enhanced resilience, and better overall well-being.

One way to cultivate positivity and gratitude is to practice daily gratitude exercises, such as keeping a gratitude journal or taking a few moments each day to reflect on the things you're thankful for. Focus on the small victories, progress, and blessings in your life, no matter how minor, and take time to appreciate the journey and the people who support you along the way.

Additionally, incorporating positive affirmations and self-talk into your daily routine can help reframe negative thought patterns and foster a more optimistic outlook. Replace self-doubt and criticism with words of encouragement, affirmation, and belief in your abilities, and notice how it impacts your mindset and motivation over time.

Conclusion

In conclusion, mindset plays a crucial role in achieving fitness success, shaping your attitudes, beliefs, and behaviors in response to challenges and setbacks. By cultivating a growth mindset focused on learning and resilience, building strong social support networks, practicing self-care, and cultivating positivity and gratitude, you can strengthen your mental resilience and unlock your full potential on your fitness journey.

Remember, your mindset is a powerful tool that can either propel you forward towards your goals or hold you back from reaching your full potential. Choose to embrace a mindset of growth, resilience, and positivity, and watch as it transforms your fitness journey and empowers you to achieve your goals with confidence and grace.

In closing, I want to thank you for joining me on this journey through "Thinner Leaner Stronger: The Simple Science of Building the Ultimate Female Body." I hope that the insights, strategies, and tools shared in this book will inspire you to cultivate a mindset of strength, resilience, and empowerment in all areas of your life.

You have everything you need within you to succeed. Now, go out there and make it happen.

Chapter 8: Beyond the Physical: Embracing the Mental and Emotional Benefits of Fitness

Welcome to Chapter 8 of "Thinner Leaner Stronger: The Simple Science of Building the Ultimate Female Body." In this chapter, we'll explore the often-overlooked mental and emotional benefits of fitness and discuss how prioritizing your mental and emotional well-being can enhance your overall quality of life and enrich your fitness journey.

The Mind-Body Connection

It's no secret that regular exercise and physical activity offer a wide range of benefits for your physical health, including improved cardiovascular health, increased strength and flexibility, and reduced risk of chronic diseases such as heart disease, diabetes, and obesity. However, what many people don't realize is that exercise also has powerful effects on your mental and emotional well-being.

The mind-body connection refers to the interrelationship between your physical health and your mental and emotional state. When you take care of your body through regular exercise, proper nutrition, and adequate rest, you also support your mental and emotional health, leading to improvements in mood, stress levels, self-esteem, and overall well-being.

Improving Mood and Mental Health

One of the most well-known mental and emotional benefits of exercise is its ability to improve mood and mental health. Physical activity has been shown to stimulate the release of endorphins – chemicals in the brain that act as natural painkillers and mood elevators – leading to feelings of happiness, relaxation, and euphoria.

Regular exercise has also been linked to reductions in symptoms of depression, anxiety, and stress, making it an effective natural treatment for mood disorders and mental health conditions. Exercise can help regulate neurotransmitters such as serotonin, dopamine, and norepinephrine, which play key roles in mood regulation and emotional well-being.

In addition to its direct effects on mood, exercise can also provide a distraction from negative thoughts and worries, promote social interaction and support networks, and foster a sense of accomplishment and mastery that boosts self-esteem and confidence.

Building Resilience and Coping Skills

In addition to improving mood and mental health, regular exercise can also help build resilience and coping skills that enhance your ability to navigate life's challenges and setbacks. Physical activity provides a safe and healthy outlet for stress and tension, allowing you to release pent-up emotions and energy in a productive way.

Engaging in regular exercise also teaches valuable skills such as goal-setting, discipline, perseverance, and resilience – qualities that can transfer to other areas of your life and help you overcome obstacles and setbacks with grace and resilience. Whether it's pushing through a tough workout, conquering a new fitness goal, or bouncing back from a setback, the mental and emotional strength you gain from exercise can empower you to face life's challenges with confidence and determination.

Boosting Self-Esteem and Confidence

Another important mental and emotional benefit of fitness is its ability to boost self-esteem and confidence. Regular exercise can improve body image, self-perception, and feelings of self-worth by helping you feel stronger, more capable, and more in control of your body and your life.

As you progress on your fitness journey and achieve your goals – whether it's lifting heavier weights, running faster, or fitting into a smaller dress size – you'll build a sense of accomplishment and pride that translates into greater confidence and self-assurance in other areas of your life. This newfound confidence can empower you to take on new challenges, pursue your passions, and live life to the fullest.

Enhancing Quality of Life

Ultimately, the mental and emotional benefits of fitness extend far beyond the physical realm, enriching your overall quality of life and well-being.

By prioritizing your mental and emotional health alongside your physical health, you can experience greater happiness, fulfillment, and vitality in all areas of your life.

So, as you embark on your fitness journey, remember to nurture your mind and spirit as well as your body. Take time to engage in activities that bring you joy, relaxation, and fulfillment, whether it's yoga, meditation, spending time in nature, or simply connecting with loved ones. By embracing the holistic benefits of fitness and wellness, you can create a life that is balanced, vibrant, and full of meaning.

Conclusion

In conclusion, fitness is not just about building a strong, healthy body – it's also about nurturing a strong, resilient mind and spirit. By prioritizing your mental and emotional well-being alongside your physical health, you can experience a wide range of benefits that enhance your overall quality of life and enrich your fitness journey.

So, as you continue on your path towards a stronger, leaner body, remember to take care of your mind and spirit as well. Cultivate self-awareness, practice self-care, and nurture positive habits and attitudes that support your mental and emotional well-being. By embracing the holistic benefits of fitness, you can create a life that is balanced, vibrant, and full of vitality.

In closing, I want to thank you for joining me on this journey through "Thinner Leaner Stronger: The Simple Science of Building the Ultimate Female Body." I hope that the insights, strategies, and inspiration shared in this book will empower you to cultivate a strong, resilient body and mind, and live a life of health, happiness, and fulfillment.

Remember, you are capable of achieving greatness in all areas of your life. Believe in yourself, stay committed to your goals, and never underestimate the power of fitness to transform your life from the inside out.

Chapter 9: Roundup: Reflecting on Your Journey and Looking Ahead

Welcome to the final chapter of "Thinner Leaner Stronger: The Simple Science of Building the Ultimate Female Body." As we come to the end of our journey together, it's time to reflect on how far you've come, celebrate your achievements, and set your sights on the road ahead. In this chapter, we'll take a comprehensive look back at the key lessons, strategies, and insights shared throughout this book, and explore how you can continue to progress and evolve on your fitness journey in the days, months, and years to come.

Reflecting on Your Journey

Take a moment to reflect on the journey you've been on since you first picked up this book. Think about where you started, the goals you set for yourself, and the obstacles you faced along the way. Consider the progress you've made, both physically and mentally, and the lessons you've learned about yourself and your body.

Celebrate your achievements, no matter how big or small, and acknowledge the hard work, dedication, and commitment that got you to where you are today. Whether you've lost weight, gained strength, improved your fitness levels, or simply developed healthier habits and routines, every step forward is a victory worth celebrating.

Key Lessons and Strategies

Throughout this book, we've covered a wide range of topics related to building a stronger, leaner body, including strength training, nutrition, supplementation, mindset, and more. As you reflect on your journey, think about the key lessons and strategies that have resonated with you and had the biggest impact on your progress.

Perhaps you've discovered the importance of progressive overload in strength training, the power of balanced nutrition for fueling your workouts and supporting recovery, or the transformative effects of cultivating a growth mindset and resilience. Maybe you've found inspiration in the stories of other women who have overcome obstacles and achieved their fitness goals, or learned practical tips and techniques for staying motivated and consistent in your training and nutrition habits.

Whatever lessons you've taken away from this book, consider how you can continue to apply them in your daily life and fitness journey moving forward. Reflect on what has worked well for you, what challenges you've encountered, and what adjustments you may need to make to keep progressing towards your goals.

Setting New Goals

With reflection comes the opportunity to set new goals and aspirations for the future. Take some time to think about what you want to achieve next on your fitness journey – whether it's building more strength, improving your endurance, mastering new skills, or reaching a specific body composition goal.

When setting new goals, remember to make them specific, measurable, achievable, relevant, and time-bound (SMART) to give yourself a clear roadmap for success. Break your goals down into smaller, more manageable milestones or action steps, and create a plan of action for achieving them.

Consider consulting with a coach, trainer, or mentor to help you set realistic goals and develop a personalized training and nutrition plan tailored to your individual needs and aspirations. Having expert guidance and support can make all the difference in staying focused, accountable, and motivated as you work towards your goals.

Embracing the Journey

As you look ahead to the future, remember to embrace the journey and enjoy the process of growth and self-discovery that comes with pursuing your fitness goals. Fitness is not just about reaching a destination or achieving a certain outcome – it's about the experiences, lessons, and personal transformations that occur along the way.

Stay open-minded, curious, and adaptable as you navigate the ups and downs of your fitness journey, and be willing to adjust your goals and plans as needed based on feedback from your body and your life circumstances. Remember that setbacks and challenges are a normal part of the process, and that each obstacle you overcome makes you stronger, more resilient, and more capable of achieving your dreams.

Gratitude and Appreciation

Finally, take a moment to express gratitude and appreciation for yourself and for the support system that has helped you along the way. Acknowledge the hard work, dedication, and perseverance you've demonstrated on your fitness journey, and celebrate the progress you've made towards becoming the best version of yourself.

Thank your friends, family, coaches, trainers, and fellow fitness enthusiasts who have supported and encouraged you on your journey, and let them know how much their support means to you. Cultivate an attitude of gratitude for the blessings and opportunities in your life, and approach each day with a sense of appreciation and abundance.

Conclusion

In conclusion, as we come to the end of "Thinner Leaner Stronger: The Simple Science of Building the Ultimate Female Body," I want to thank you for joining me on this journey of self-discovery, growth, and empowerment. Whether you're just starting out on your fitness journey or you're a seasoned athlete, I hope that the insights, strategies, and inspiration shared in this book have empowered you to take control of your health, fitness, and happiness.

Remember, your fitness journey is a marathon, not a sprint – it's a lifelong process of growth and self-improvement that unfolds one step at a time. Stay committed to your goals, stay curious, and stay open to new possibilities and experiences along the way.

No matter where your journey takes you, know that you have everything you need within you to succeed. Believe in yourself, trust in your abilities, and never underestimate the power of persistence, resilience, and determination to help you achieve your dreams.

Thank you for allowing me to be a part of your journey, and I wish you continued success, happiness, and fulfillment in all your endeavors.

In conclusion, "Thinner Leaner Stronger: The Simple Science of Building the Ultimate Female Body" has been a journey of empowerment, self-discovery, and transformation. Throughout this book, we've explored the principles and practices of strength training, nutrition, mindset, and holistic wellness, with the goal of empowering you to take control of your health, fitness, and happiness.

As we close this chapter, I want to leave you with a few key takeaways to carry forward on your journey:

1. **Believe in Yourself:** You are capable of achieving greatness in all areas of your life. Believe in your abilities, trust in your potential, and never underestimate the power of persistence, resilience, and determination to help you achieve your dreams.

2. **Prioritize Your Health:** Your health is your greatest asset, and investing in it is the most important investment you can make. Prioritize your physical, mental, and emotional well-being by adopting healthy habits, nourishing your body with nutritious foods, and staying active and engaged in activities that bring you joy and fulfillment.

3. **Embrace the Journey:** Fitness is not just about reaching a destination or achieving a certain outcome – it's about the experiences, lessons, and personal transformations that occur along the way. Embrace the journey, stay open-minded and adaptable, and enjoy the process of growth and self-discovery that comes with pursuing your goals.

4. **Cultivate Gratitude:** Cultivate an attitude of gratitude for the blessings and opportunities in your life, and approach each day with a sense of appreciation and abundance. Express gratitude for yourself and for the support system that has helped you along the way, and let those around you know how much their support means to you.

5. **Stay Curious and Open-Minded:** Keep an open mind, stay curious, and be willing to explore new possibilities and experiences on your journey.

Continuously seek out opportunities for learning and growth, and be willing to adapt and evolve as you discover what works best for you and your body.

As you continue on your journey of health, fitness, and self-discovery, remember that you have everything you need within you to succeed. Trust in yourself, believe in your potential, and never forget the power of persistence, resilience, and determination to help you achieve your goals.

Thank you for allowing me to be a part of your journey, and I wish you continued success, happiness, and fulfillment in all your endeavors.